THE SUPER EASY PLANT BASED DIET COOKBOOK

Easy and affordable recipes that beginners and advanced can cook. Reset metabolism, heal your body and regain confidence.

Ursa Males

TABLE OF CONTENTS

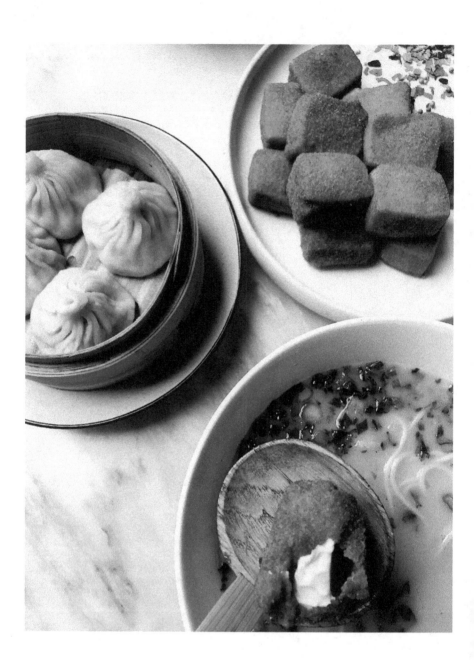

BREAKFAST

1. Keto Porridge

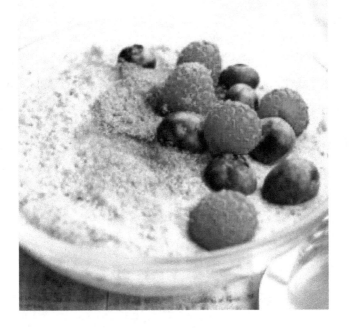

Preparation time: 15 minutes

Cooking time: 10 minutes

Servings: 1

Ingredients:

- ½ tsp vanilla extract
- ¼ tsp granulated stevia
- 1 tbsp chia seeds
- 1 tbsp flaxseed meal

- 2 tbsp unsweetened shredded coconut
- 2 tbsp almond flour
- 2 tbsp hemp hearts
- ½ cup of water
- Pinch of salt

Directions:

1. Add all fixings except vanilla extract to a saucepan and heat over low heat until thickened. Stir well and serve warm.

Nutrition: Calories 370Fat 30.2 g Carbohydrates 12.8 g Protein 13.5 g

2. Chia Seed Pudding

Preparation time: 15 minutes

Cooking time: 0 minutes

Servings: 4

Ingredients:

- ¼ tsp. cinnamon
- 15 drops liquid stevia
- ½ tsp. vanilla extract
- ½ cup chia seeds
- 2 cups unsweetened coconut milk

Directions:

1. Add all ingredients into the glass jar and mix well. Close jar with lid and place in the refrigerator for 4 hours. Serve chilled and enjoy.

Nutrition: Calories 347 Fat 33.2 g Carbohydrates 9.8 g Protein 5.9 g

3. Vegan Zoodles

Preparation time: 15 minutes

Cooking time: 10 minutes

Servings: 4

Ingredients:

- 4 small zucchinis, spiralized into noodles
- 3 tbsp vegetable stock
- 1 cup red pepper, diced
- 1/2 cup onion, diced
- 3/4 cup nutritional yeast
- 1 tbsp garlic powder
- Pepper
- Salt

Directions:

1. Add zucchini noodles, red pepper, and onion in a pan with vegetable stock and cook over medium heat for a few minutes.
2. Add nutritional yeast and garlic powder and cook for few minutes until creamy—season with pepper and salt. Stir well and serve.

Nutrition: Calories 71Fat 0.9 g Carbohydrates 12.1 g

Protein 5.7 g

4. Avocado Tofu Scramble

Preparation time: 15 minutes

Cooking time: 7 minutes

Servings: 1

Ingredients:

- 1 tbsp fresh parsley, chopped
- ½ medium avocado
- ½ block firm tofu drained and crumbled
- ½ cup bell pepper, chopped
- ½ cup onion, chopped
- 1 tsp olive oil
- 1 tbsp water
- ¼ tsp cumin
- ¼ tsp garlic powder
- ¼ tsp paprika
- ¼ tsp turmeric
- 1 tbsp nutritional yeast
- Pepper
- Salt

Directions:

1. In a bowl, mix nut yeast, water, and spices. Put it separately. Now heat the olive oil to the pan over medium heat.

2. Add onion and bell pepper and sauté for 5 minutes. Add crumbled tofu and nutritional yeast to the pan and sauté for 2 minutes. Top with parsley and avocado. Serve and enjoy.

Nutrition: Calories 164Fat 9.7 g Carbohydrates 15 g Protein 7.4 g

5. Tofu Fries

Preparation time: 15 minutes

Cooking time: 20 minutes

Servings: 4

Ingredients:

- 15 oz firm tofu, drained, pressed, and cut into long strips
- ¼ tsp garlic powder
- ¼ tsp onion powder
- ¼ tsp cayenne pepper
- ¼ tsp paprika
- ½ tsp oregano
- ½ tsp basil
- 2 tbsp olive oil
- Pepper
- Salt

Directions:

1. Warm oven to 375 F. Add all ingredients into the large mixing bowl and toss well. Place marinated tofu strips on a baking tray and bake in a preheated oven for 20 minutes.

2. Turn tofu strips to the other side and bake for another 20 minutes. Serve and enjoy.

Nutrition: Calories 137Fat 11.5 g Carbohydrates 2.3 g Protein 8.8 g

6. Chia Raspberry Pudding Shots

Preparation time: 1 hour & 15 minutes

Cooking time: 0 minutes

Servings: 4

Ingredients:

- ½ cup raspberries
- 10 drops liquid stevia
- 1 tbsp unsweetened cocoa powder
- ¼ cup unsweetened almond milk
- ½ cup unsweetened coconut milk
- ¼ cup chia seeds

Directions:

1. Add all ingredients into the glass jar and stir well to combine. Pour pudding mixture into the shot glasses and place in the refrigerator for 1 hour. Serve chilled and enjoy.

Nutrition: Calories 117Fat 10 g Carbohydrates 5.9 g Protein 2.7 g

7. <u>Chia-Almond Pudding</u>

Preparation time: 60 minutes

Cooking time: 0 minutes

Servings: 2

Ingredients:

- ½ tsp vanilla extract
- ¼ tsp almond extract
- 2 tbsp ground almonds
- 1 ½ cups unsweetened almond milk
- ¼ cup chia seeds

Directions:

1. Add chia seeds in almond milk and soak for 1 hour. Add chia seed and almond milk into the blender.
2. Add remaining ingredients to the blender and blend until smooth and creamy. Serve and enjoy.

Nutrition: Calories 138Fat 10.2 g Carbohydrates 6 g Protein 5.1 g

8. Fresh Berries with Cream

Preparation time: 15 minutes

Cooking time: 0 minutes

Servings: 1

Ingredients:

- 1/2 cup coconut cream
- 1 oz strawberries
- 1 oz raspberries
- 1/4 tsp vanilla extract

Directions:

1. Add all fixings into the blender and blend until smooth. Pour in serving bowl and top with fresh berries. Serve and enjoy.

Nutrition: Calories 303Fat 28.9 g Carbohydrates 12 g Protein 3.3 g

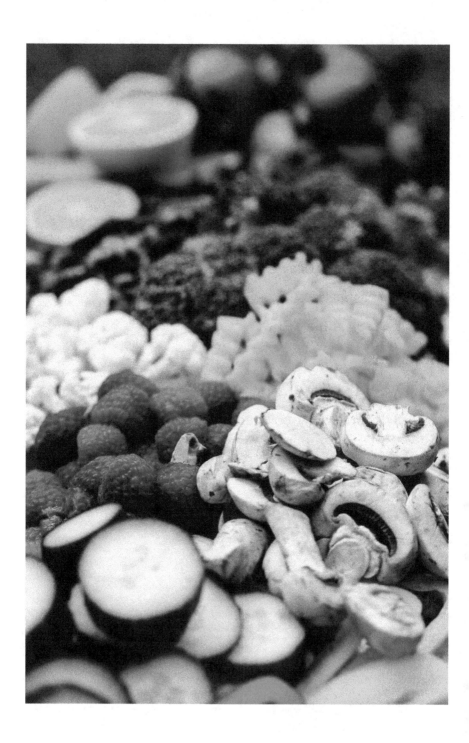

LUNCH

9. Spicy Hummus Quesadillas

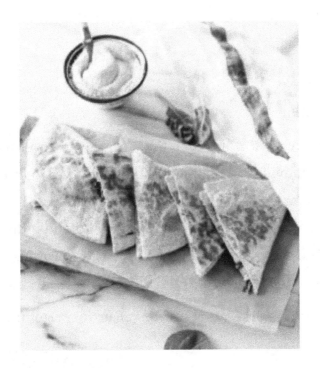

Preparation time: 5 minutes

Cooking time: 15 minutes

Servings: 4

Ingredients:

- 4 x 8" whole grain tortilla
- 1 cup hummus

- Your choice of fillings: spinach, sundried tomatoes, olives, etc.
- Extra-virgin olive oil for brushing

To serve:

- Extra hummus
- Hot sauce
- Pesto

Directions:

1. Put your tortillas on a flat surface and cover each with hummus. Add the fillings, then fold over to form a half-moon shape.
2. Pop a skillet over medium heat and add a drop of oil. Add the quesadillas and flip when browned. Repeat with the remaining quesadillas, then serve and enjoy.

Nutrition: Calories: 256Carbs: 25gFat: 12gProtein: 7g

10. Quinoa Lentil Burger

Preparation time: 5 minutes

Cooking time: 25 minutes

Servings: 4

Ingredients:

- 1 tablespoon + 2 teaspoons of olive oil
- ¼ cup red onion, diced
- 1 cup quinoa, cooked
- 1 cup cooked drained brown lentils
- 1 x 4 oz. green chilies, diced
- 1/3 cup oats, rolled
- ¼ cup flour
- 2 teaspoons corn starch
- ¼ cup panko breadcrumbs, whole-wheat
- ¼ teaspoon garlic powder
- ½ teaspoon cumin
- Paprika,1 teaspoon
- Salt and pepper
- 2 tablespoons Dijon mustard
- 3 teaspoons honey

Directions:

1. Put 2 teaspoons olive oil into your skillet over medium heat. Add the onion and cook for five minutes until soft. Grab a small bowl and add the honey and Dijon mustard.

2. Grab a large bowl and add the burger ingredients; stir well. Form into 4 patties with your hands. Put a tablespoon of oil into your skillet over medium heat.

3. Add the patties and cook for 10 minutes on each side. Serve with the honey mustard and enjoy!

Nutrition: Calories: 268Carbs: 33gFat: 8gProtein: 10g

11. **Spanish Vegetable Paella**

Preparation time: 15 minutes

Cooking time: 1 hour & 30 minutes

Servings: 6

Ingredients:

- 3 tablespoons virgin olive oil, divided
- 1 medium chopped fine yellow onion
- 1 ½ teaspoon fine sea salt, divided
- 6 garlic cloves, minced or pressed
- 2 teaspoons smoked paprika
- 15 oz. can dice tomatoes, drained
- 2 cups short-grain brown rice
- 15 oz. can garbanzo beans, rinsed & drained
- 3 cups vegetable broth
- 1/3 cup dry white wine/vegetable broth
- ½ teaspoon saffron threads, crumbled (optional)
- 14 oz. can quarter artichokes
- 2 red bell peppers, sliced into long, ½"-wide strips
- ½ cup Kalamata olives pitted and halved
- ¼ tsp ground black pepper
- ¼ cup chopped fresh parsley, + about 1 tablespoon more for garnish
- 2 tablespoons lemon juice

- Lemon wedges for garnish
- ½ cup frozen peas

Directions:

1. Preheat the oven to 350°F. Put 2 tablespoons of oil into your skillet and pop over medium heat. Add the onion and cook for five minutes until soft.

2. Add salt, garlic, and paprika—Cook for 30 seconds. Add the tomatoes, stir through and cook for 2 minutes. Add the rice, stir through, and cook again for a minute.

3. Add the garbanzo beans, broth, wine or stock, saffron, and salt, and bring to a boil. Cover and pop into the oven within 40 minutes until the rice has been absorbed. Line a baking sheet with parchment paper.

4. Grab a large bowl and add the artichoke, peppers, olives, 1 tablespoon olive oil, ½ Teaspoon of salt, and black pepper to taste. Toss to combine, then spread over the prepared baking sheet.

5. Pop into the oven and cook within 30 minutes. Remove from the oven and leave to cool slightly. Add the parsley, lemon juice, and seasoning as required. Toss.

6. Pop the rice onto a stove, turn up the heat and bake the rice for five minutes. Garnish and serve with the veggies.

Nutrition: Calories: 437Carbs: 60gFat: 16gProtein: 10g

12.   Tex-Mex Tofu & Beans

Preparation time: 25 minutes

Cooking time: 12 minutes

Servings: 2

Ingredients:

- 1 cup dry black beans
- 1 cup dry brown rice
- 1 14-oz. package firm tofu, drained
- 2 tbsp. olive oil
- 1 small purple onion, diced
- 1 medium avocado, pitted, peeled
- 1 garlic clove, minced
- 1 tbsp. lime juice
- 2 tsp. cumin
- 2 tsp. paprika
- 1 tsp. chili powder
- Salt and pepper to taste

Directions:

1. Cut the tofu into ½-inch cubes. Heat the olive oil in a skillet. Put the diced onions and cook until soft, for about 5 minutes.

2. Add the tofu and cook an additional 2 minutes, flipping the cubes frequently. Meanwhile, cut the avocado into thin slices and set aside.

3. Lower the heat and add in the garlic, cumin, and cooked black beans. Stir until everything is incorporated thoroughly, and then cook for an additional 5 minutes.

4. Add the remaining spices and lime juice to the mixture in the skillet. Mix thoroughly and remove the skillet from the heat.

5. Serve the Tex-Mex tofu and beans with a scoop of rice and garnish with the fresh avocado. Enjoy immediately, or store the rice, avocado, and tofu mixture separately.

Nutrition: Calories: 315Carbs: 27.8 g Fat: 17 g Protein: 12.7 g.

13. **Spaghetti Squash Burrito Bowl**

Preparation time: 5 minutes

Cooking time: 60 minutes

Servings: 4

Ingredients:

- 2 x 2 lb. spaghetti squash, halved and seeds removed
- 2 tablespoons olive oil
- Salt
- ground black pepper, to taste
- For the cabbage and black bean slaw:
- 2 cups purple cabbage, sliced thinly
- 15 oz. can black beans
- 2 tablespoons fresh lime juice
- 1 red bell pepper, sliced
- 1/3 cup chopped green onions
- 1/3 cup chopped fresh cilantro
- 1 teaspoon olive oil
- ¼ teaspoon salt

For the avocado salsa Verde:

- ¾ cup mild salsa Verde
- 1/3 cup fresh cilantro
- 1 avocado, diced
- 1 tbsp. fresh lime juice

- 1 chopped garlic clove

To garnish:

- Chopped fresh cilantro
- Crumbled feta
- Seasoned toasted pepitas

Directions:

1. Preheat your oven to 400°F and line a baking sheet with parchment paper. Place the spaghetti squash on top and drizzle with olive oil. Rub into the flesh
2. Sprinkle with salt and pepper and turn, so the cut sides are down. Roast for 40-60 minutes until soft.
3. Meanwhile, grab a medium bowl and add all the ingredients for the cabbage and black bean slaw. Stir well, then pop to one side.
4. Grab your blender, then add the salsa Verde ingredients. Whizz until smooth. Remove squash from the oven and use the fork to fluff up.
5. Divide between your serving bowls, then top with the slaw and the avocado salsa Verde. Top with the topping of your choice, then serve and enjoy.

Nutrition: Calories: 301Carbs: 21gFat: 17gProtein: 8g

14. No-Egg Salad

Preparation time: 15 minutes

Cooking time: 0 minutes

Servings: 6

Ingredients:

- 1 (13-ounce) package firm tofu
- 1 celery stalk, finely chopped
- ¼ cup chives, finely chopped
- 1 tablespoon nutritional yeast
- 1 teaspoon turmeric
- ¼ teaspoon garlic powder
- ¼ teaspoon celery seed (optional)
- ½ teaspoon black salt (Kala namak)
- 2 tablespoon vegan mayonnaise
- 2 tablespoon dill pickle relish
- 1 tablespoon Dijon mustard
- 1 tablespoon fresh lemon juice
- Salt
- Freshly ground black pepper

Directions:

1. Crumble the tofu into a medium bowl with your hands. Then add the celery, chives, nutritional yeast, turmeric, garlic powder, celery seed (if using), and black salt and mix well.

2. In a small measuring cup or bowl, combine the vegan mayo, relish, mustard, and lemon juice to make a dressing. Put the dressing over the tofu batter and stir until everything is well combined.

3. Taste and season with salt and pepper, if desired. Enjoy.

Nutrition: Calories: 87Fat: 5gCarbohydrate: 5gProtein: 7g

15. Chickpea No Tuna Salad

Preparation time: 5 minutes

Cooking time: 0 minutes

Servings: 3

Ingredients:

- 1 (14-ounce) can chickpeas, drained and rinsed
- 2 celery stalks, finely chopped
- 2 scallions, coarsely chopped
- 2 tablespoons vegan mayonnaise
- Juice of ½ lemon
- 2 heaping teaspoons capers and brine
- 1 teaspoon dried dill or 1 handful fresh dill, chopped
- ½ teaspoon Dijon mustard
- ¼ teaspoon kelp flakes
- ¼ to ½ teaspoon salt
- Freshly ground black pepper

Directions:

1. In a medium bowl, combine the chickpeas, celery, scallions, mayo, lemon juice, capers, dill, mustard, kelp flakes, salt, and pepper.
2. Mix and mash everything together using a potato masher. Taste then flavor with additional salt, pepper,

or lemon, if desired. Enjoy on its own, on top of a romaine or endive leaf, or with rice cakes.

Nutrition: Calories: 193Fat: 4gCarbohydrate: 33g Protein: 7g

DINNER

16.   <u>Tomato, Kale, and White Bean Skillet</u>

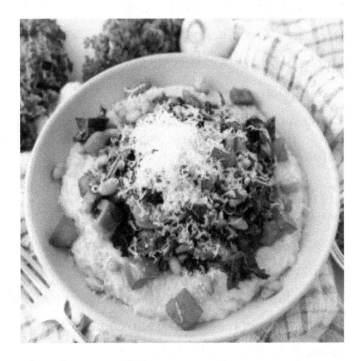

Preparation time: 10 minutes

Cooking time: 10 minutes

Servings: 4

Ingredients:

- 30 ounces cooked cannellini beans
- 3 1/2 ounces sun-dried tomatoes, chopped, packed in oil

- 6 ounces kale, chopped
- 1 teaspoon minced garlic
- 1/4 teaspoon ground black pepper
- 1/4 teaspoon salt
- 1/2 tablespoon dried basil
- 1/8 teaspoon red pepper flakes
- 1 tablespoon apple cider vinegar
- 1 tablespoon olive oil
- 2 tablespoons oil from sun-dried tomatoes

Directions:

1. Prepare the dressing and for this, place basil, black pepper, salt, vinegar, and red pepper flakes in a small bowl, add oil from sun-dried tomatoes and whisk until combined.

2. Take a skillet pan, place it over medium heat, add olive oil and when hot, add garlic and cook for 1 minute until fragrant.

3. Add kale, splash with some water and cook for 3 minutes until kale leaves have wilted. Add tomatoes and beans, stir well and cook for 3 minutes until heated.

4. Remove pan from heat, drizzle with the prepared dressing, toss until mixed and serve.

Nutrition: Calories: 264 Fat: 12 g Carbs: 38 g Protein: 9 g

17. Chard Wraps with Millet

Preparation time: 25 minutes

Cooking time: 0 minute

Servings: 4

Ingredients:

- 1 carrot, cut into ribbons
- 1/2 cup millet, cooked
- 1/2 of a large cucumber, cut into ribbons
- 1/2 cup chickpeas, cooked
- 1 cup sliced cabbage
- 1/3 cup hummus
- Mint leaves as needed for topping
- Hemp seeds as needed for topping
- 1 bunch of Swiss rainbow chard

Directions:

1. Spread hummus on one side of chard, place some of millet, vegetables, and chickpeas on it, sprinkle with some mint leaves and hemp seeds and wrap it like a burrito. Serve straight away.

Nutrition: Calories: 152 Fat: 4.5 g Carbs: 25 g Protein: 3.5 g

18. <u>Stuffed Peppers with Kidney Beans</u>

Preparation time: 5 minutes

Cooking time: 35 minutes

Servings: 4

Ingredients:

- 3 1/2 ounces cooked kidney beans
- 1 big tomato, diced
- 3 1/2 ounces sweet corn, canned
- 2 medium bell peppers, deseeded, halved
- ½ of medium red onion, peeled, diced
- 1 teaspoon garlic powder
- 1/3 teaspoon ground black pepper
- 2/3 teaspoon salt
- ½ teaspoon dried basil
- 3 teaspoons parsley
- ½ teaspoon dried thyme
- 3 tablespoons cashew
- 1 teaspoon olive oil

Directions:

1. Switch on the oven, then set it to 400 degrees F and let it preheat. Take a large skillet pan, place it over medium heat, add oil and when hot, add onion and cook for 2 minutes until translucent.

2. Add beans, tomatoes, and corn, stir in garlic and cashews and cook for 5 minutes.
3. Stir in salt, black pepper, parsley, basil, and thyme, remove the pan from heat and evenly divide the mixture between bell peppers. Bake the peppers for 25 minutes until tender, then top with parsley and serve.

Nutrition: Calories: 139 Fat: 1.6 g Carbs: 18 g Protein: 5.1 g

19. Summer Harvest Pizza

Preparation Time: 20 minutes

Cooking Time: 15 minutes

Servings: 2

Ingredients:

- 1 lavash flatbread, whole grain
- 4 tbsp feta spread, store-bought
- ½ cup cheddar cheese, shredded
- ½ cup corn kernels, cooked
- ½ cup beans, cooked
- ½ cup fire-roasted red peppers, chopped

Directions:

1. Preheat oven to 350°F. Cut Lavash into two halves. Bake crusts on a pan in the oven for 5 minutes.
2. Spread feta spread on both crusts. Top with remaining ingredients. Bake for another 10 minutes.

Nutrition: Calories 230 Carbohydrates 23 g Fats 15 g Protein 11 g

20. <u>Whole Wheat Pizza with Summer Produce</u>

Preparation Time: 15 minutes

Cooking Time: 15 minutes

Servings: 2

Ingredients:

- 1-pound whole wheat pizza dough
- 4 ounces goat cheese
- 2/3 cup blueberries
- 2 ears corn, husked
- 2 yellow squash, sliced
- 2 tbsp olive oil

Directions:

1. Preheat the oven to 450°F. Roll the dough out to make a pizza crust.
2. Crumble the cheese on the crust. Spread remaining ingredients, then drizzle with olive oil.

3. Bake for about 15 minutes. Serve.

Nutrition: Calories 470 Carbohydrates 66 g Fats 18 g Protein 17 g

21. <u>Tempeh Tikka Masala</u>

Preparation time: 15 minutes

Cooking time: 20 minutes

Servings: 3

Ingredients:

Tempeh:

- ½ tsp sea salt

1 tsp of the following:

- garam masala
- ginger, ground
- cumin, ground
- 2 tsp apple cider vinegar
- ½ cup vegan yogurt
- 8 oz. tempeh, cubed

Tikka Masala Sauce:

- 2 cups frozen peas

1 cup of the following:

- full-fat coconut milk
- tomato sauce
- ¼ tsp turmeric
- ½ tsp sea salt
- 1 onion, chopped

1 tsp of the following:

- chili powder
- garam masala
- 1/4 cup ginger, freshly grated
- 3 cloves garlic, minced
- 1 tbsp. coconut oil

Directions:

1. Begin with making the tempeh by combining sea salt, garam masala, ginger, cumin, vinegar, and yogurt in a bowl. Add tempeh to the bowl and coat well; cover the bowl and refrigerate for 60 minutes.
2. In a pan big enough for 3 servings, add some coconut oil to heat using the medium setting, and begin preparing the sauce.
3. Sauté in the ginger, garlic, and onion for 5 minutes or until fragrant. Add the garam masala, chili powder, sea salt, and turmeric and combine well.
4. Add the frozen peas, coconut, milk, tomato sauce, and tempeh, reducing the heat to medium. Simmer within 15 minutes

5. Remove from the heat and serve with cauliflower rice.

Nutrition: Calories: 430 Carbohydrates: 39 g Proteins: 21 g Fats: 23 g

22. <u>Caprice Casserole</u>

Preparation time: 15 minutes

Cooking time: 37 minutes

Servings: 3

Ingredients:

Tempeh:

- ¼ cup basil, chopped
- 1 tomato, big
- ¼ tsp pepper
- ½ tsp salt

1 tbsp. of the following:

- nutritional yeast
- tahini
- 1 clove garlic
- 14 oz. tofu, extra firm, drained
- 6 cups marinara sauce
- 10 oz. vegetable noodles

Directions:

1. Set the oven to 350 heat setting. Cut the tofu into 4 slabs and remove excess moisture by gently squeezing each slab with a paper towel.

2. In a food processor, add garlic and chop, then scrape garlic from the sides to ensure it will be thoroughly mixed.

3. Add pepper, salt, yeast, tahini, and tofu to the food processor and pulse for 15 to 20 seconds until fully combined and forming a paste.

4. In an oven-safe dish, spread ½ cup of the marinara sauce across the bottom. Divide the vegetable noodles in half, break the noodles, and layer them on top of the sauce.

5. Put another layer of sauce over your noodles. Add the remaining noodles and coat the top with remaining sauce.

6. Using the tofu mixture from the food processor, form little patties about ½ thick and place on top of the sauce, filling up the dish.

7. Cover the baking container with aluminum foil and bake for 20 minutes. Uncover and bake again within 15 minutes.

8. Remove from the oven and set the oven to broil. Place the tomato slices on top of tofu mixture and broil for 2 minutes or until the tofu is lightly toasted.

9. Garnish with basil. Serve warm and enjoy.

Nutrition: Calories: 642 Carbohydrates: 88.6 g Proteins: 25.1 g Fats: 5.1 g

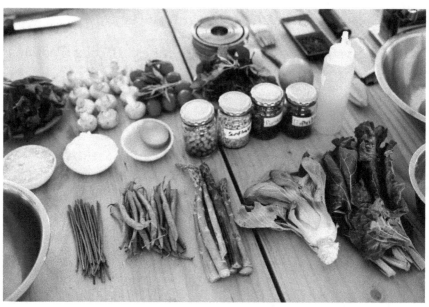

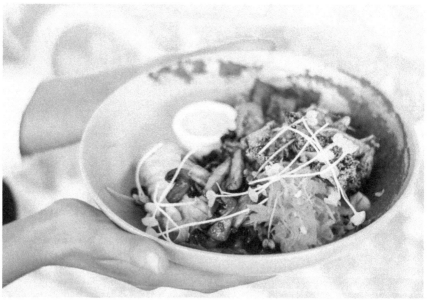

SNACKS

23. Lentil Cakes

Preparation time: 10 minutes

Cooking time: 10 minutes

Servings: 8

Ingredients:

- 2 teaspoons basil, dried
- 1 cup chopped yellow onion
- 1 cup leeks, chopped
- 1 cup canned red lentils, drained and rinsed
- 1 teaspoon coriander, ground
- ¼ cup chopped parsley
- 1 tablespoon curry powder
- ¼ cup chopped cilantro
- 2 tablespoons coconut flour
- 1 tablespoon olive oil

Directions:

1. Put the lentils in your bowl and mash them well using a potato masher. Add the basil, onion and the other ingredients except the oil and stir. Shape medium cakes out of this mix.

2. Warm-up a pan with the oil over medium-high heat, add the cakes and cook them for about 5 minutes on each side. Serve warm.

Nutrition: Calories 142Fat 4gCarbs 8gProtein 4.4g

24.   Tomato and Avocado Salsa

Preparation time: 10 minutes

Cooking time: 0 minutes

Servings: 6

Ingredients:

- 3 cups chopped tomatoes
- 1 cup avocado, peeled, pitted and chopped
- 1 tablespoon black olives, pitted and sliced
- 1 red onion, chopped
- 2 teaspoons capers
- 3 garlic cloves, minced
- 2 teaspoons balsamic vinegar
- 1 tablespoon chopped basil
- A pinch of salt and black pepper

Directions:

1. Mix the tomatoes with the avocado, olives and the other ingredients in a bowl and toss. Serve.

Nutrition: Calories 201Fat 4.9gCarbs 8gProtein 6g

25. **Pea Dip**

Preparation time: 10 minutes

Cooking time: 0 minutes

Servings: 8

Ingredients:

- 2 cups canned black-eyed peas, drained and rinsed
- ½ teaspoon chili powder
- ½ cup coconut cream
- A pinch of salt and black pepper
- ½ teaspoon garlic powder
- 1 teaspoon Italian seasoning
- ½ teaspoon chili sauce
- 1 teaspoon hot paprika

Directions:

1. In a blender, mix the peas with the chili powder, cream and the other ingredients, blend and serve.

Nutrition: Calories 127Fat 5gCarbs 18gProtein 8g

26. Chili Walnuts

Preparation time: 10 minutes

Cooking time: 10 minutes

Servings: 4

Ingredients:

- ½ teaspoon chili flakes
- ½ teaspoon curry powder
- ½ teaspoon hot paprika
- A pinch of cayenne pepper
- 14 ounces walnuts
- 2 teaspoons avocado oil

Directions:

1. Put the walnuts on your lined baking sheet, add the chili and the other ingredients, toss, introduce in the oven and bake at 400 degrees F for 10 minutes.
2. Divide the mix into bowls and serve as a snack.

Nutrition: Calories 204Fat 3.2gCarbs 7.4gProtein 7g

27. Seed and Apricot Bowls

Preparation time: 10 minutes

Cooking time: 10 minutes

Servings: 4

Ingredients:

- 6 ounces apricots, dried
- 1 cup sunflower seeds
- 2 tablespoons coconut, shredded
- 1 tablespoon sesame seeds
- 1 tablespoon avocado oil
- 3 tablespoons hemp seeds
- 1 tablespoon chia seeds

Directions:

1. Spread the apricots, seeds and the other ingredients on a lined baking sheet, toss and cook at 430 degrees F for 10 minutes.
2. Cool down, divide into bowls and serve as a snack.

Nutrition: Calories 200Fat 4.3gCarbs 8gProtein 5g

VEGETABLES

28. Roasted Brussels Sprouts

Preparation Time: 30 minutes

Cooking Time: 20 minutes

Servings: 4

Ingredients:

- 1 lb. Brussels sprouts, sliced in half
- 1 shallot, chopped
- 1 tablespoon olive oil
- Salt and pepper to taste
- 2 teaspoons balsamic vinegar
- ¼ cup pomegranate seeds
- ¼ cup goat cheese, crumbled

Direction:

1. Preheat your oven to 400 degrees F.
2. Coat the Brussels sprouts with oil.
3. Sprinkle with salt and pepper.
4. Transfer to a baking pan.
5. Roast in the oven for 20 minutes.

6. Drizzle with the vinegar.

7. Sprinkle with the seeds and cheese before serving.

Nutrition: 117 Calories 4.8g Fiber 5.8g Protein

29. Brussels Sprouts & Cranberries

Preparation Time: 10 minutes

Cooking Time: 0 minute

Servings: 6

Ingredients:

- 3 tablespoons lemon juice
- ¼ cup olive oil
- Salt and pepper to taste
- 1 lb. Brussels sprouts, sliced thinly
- ¼ cup dried cranberries, chopped
- ½ cup pecans, toasted and chopped
- ½ cup Parmesan cheese, shaved

Direction

1. Mix the lemon juice, olive oil, salt and pepper in a bowl.
2. Toss the Brussels sprouts, cranberries and pecans in this mixture.
3. Sprinkle the Parmesan cheese on top.

Nutrition: 245 Calories 6.4g Protein 5g Fiber

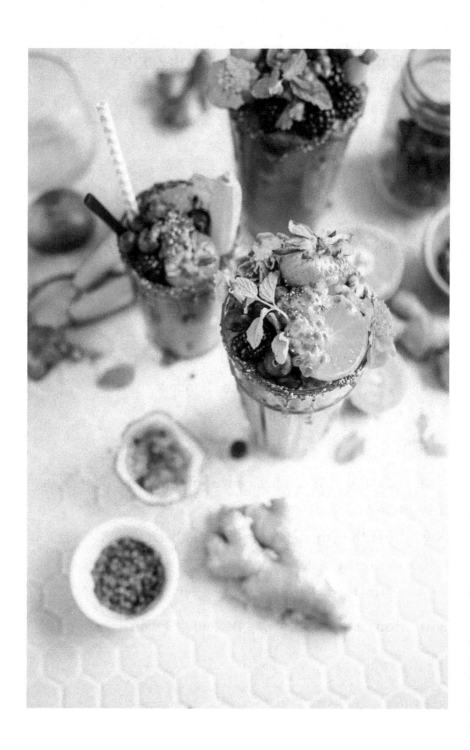

SALAD

30. Arugula Salad

Preparation Time: 15 minutes

Cooking Time: 0 minute

Servings: 4

Ingredients:

- 6 cups fresh arugula leaves
- 2 cups radicchio, chopped
- ¼ cup low-fat balsamic vinaigrette
- ¼ cup pine nuts, toasted and chopped

Instructions:

1. Arrange the arugula leaves in a serving bowl.
2. Sprinkle the radicchio on top.
3. Drizzle with the vinaigrette.
4. Sprinkle the pine nuts on top.

Nutrition: Calories 85 Fat 6.6 g Saturated fat 0.5 Carbohydrates 5.1 g Fiber 1 g Protein 2.2 g

31. **Mediterranean Salad**

Preparation Time: 20 minutes

Cooking Time: 5 minutes

Servings: 2

Ingredients:

- 2 teaspoons balsamic vinegar
- 1 tablespoon basil pesto
- 1 cup lettuce
- ¼ cup broccoli florets, chopped
- ½ cup zucchini, chopped
- ¼ cup tomato, chopped
- ¼ cup yellow bell pepper, chopped
- 2 tablespoons feta cheese, crumbled

Instructions:

1. Arrange the lettuce on a serving platter.
2. Top with the broccoli, zucchini, tomato and bell pepper.
3. In a bowl, mix the vinegar and pesto.
4. Drizzle the dressing on top.

5. Sprinkle the feta cheese and serve.

Nutrition: Calories 100 Fat 6 g Saturated fat 1 g Carbohydrates 7 g Protein 4 g

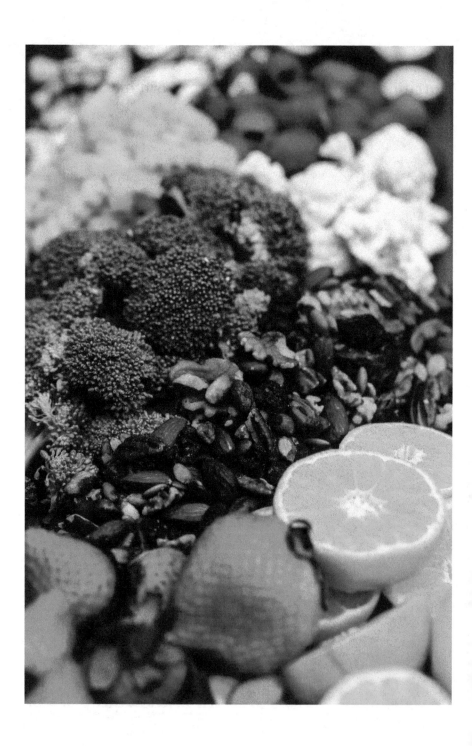

GRAINS

32. Black Bean Stuffed Sweet Potatoes

Preparation Time: 5 minutes

Cooking Time: 1 hour

Servings: 4

Ingredients:

- 4 sweet potatoes
- 15 oz. cooked black beans
- ½ tsp. ground black pepper
- ½ red onion, peeled, diced
- ½ tsp. sea salt
- ¼ tsp. onion powder
- ¼ tsp. garlic powder
- ¼ tsp. red chili powder
- ¼ tsp. cumin
- 1 tsp. lime juice
- 1 ½ tbsps. olive oil
- ½ c. cashew cream sauce

Directions:

1. Spread sweet potatoes on a baking tray greased with foil and bake for 65 minutes at 350 degrees' f until tender.

2. Meanwhile, prepare the sauce, and for this, whisk together the cream sauce, black pepper, and lime juice until combined, set aside until required.

3. When 10 minutes of the baking time of potatoes are left, heat a skillet pan with oil. Add in onion to cook until golden for 5 minutes.

4. Then stir in spice, cook for another 3 minutes, stir in bean until combined and cook for 5 minutes until hot.

5. Let roasted sweet potatoes cool for 10 minutes, then cut them open, mash the flesh and top with bean mixture, cilantro and avocado, and then drizzle with cream sauce.

6. Serve straight away.

Nutrition: Calories: 387, Fat: 16.1 g, Carbs: 53 g, Protein: 10.4 g

33. Black Bean and Quinoa Salad

Preparation Time: 10 minutes

Cooking Time: 0 minute

Servings: 10

Ingredients:

- 15 oz. cooked black beans
- 1 chopped red bell pepper, cored
- 1 c. quinoa, cooked
- 1 cored green bell pepper, chopped
- ½ c. vegan feta cheese, crumbled

Directions:

1. In a bowl, set in all ingredients, except for cheese, and stir until incorporated.
2. Top the salad with cheese and serve straight away.

Nutrition: Calories: 64, Fat: 1 g, Carbs: 8 g, Protein: 3 g

LEGUMES

34. Brown Lentil Bowl

Preparation Time: 10 minutes

Cooking Time: 10 minutes

Servings: 4

Ingredients:

- 1 cup brown lentils, soaked overnight and drained
- 3 cups water
- 2 cups brown rice, cooked
- 1 zucchini, diced
- 1 red onion, chopped
- 1 teaspoon garlic, minced
- 1 cucumber, sliced
- 1 bell pepper, sliced
- 4 tablespoons olive oil
- 1 tablespoon rice vinegar
- 2 tablespoons lemon juice
- 2 tablespoons soy sauce
- 1/2 teaspoon dried oregano
- 1/2 teaspoon ground cumin
- Sea salt and ground black pepper, to taste

- 2 cups arugula
- 2 cups Romaine lettuce, torn into pieces

Directions

1. Add the brown lentils and water to a saucepan and bring to a boil over high heat. Then, turn the heat to a simmer and continue to cook for 20 minutes or until tender.
2. Place the lentils in a salad bowl and let them cool completely.
3. Add in the remaining ingredients and toss to combine well. Serve at room temperature or well-chilled. Bon appétit!

Nutrition: Calories: 452; Fat: 16.6g; Carbs: 61.7g; Protein: 16.4g

BREAD & PIZZA

35. <u>Banana Zucchini Bread</u>

Preparation Time: 10 Minutes

Cooking Time: 45 Minutes

Servings: 12

Ingredients:

- Eggs – 4
- Cinnamon – 1 tablespoon.
- Baking soda – 3/4 teaspoon.
- Coconut flour – 1/2 cup
- Coconut oil – 1 tablespoon.
- Banana – 1, mashed
- Stevia – 1 teaspoon.
- Zucchini – 1 cup, shredded and squeezed out all liquid
- Walnuts – 1/2 cup, chopped
- Apple cider vinegar – 1 teaspoon.
- Nutmeg – 1/2 teaspoon.
- Salt – 1/2 teaspoon.

Directions:

1. Preheat the oven to 350 F. Grease loaf pan with oil and set aside. In a large bowl, whisk together egg, banana, oil, and stevia.

2. Add all dry Ingredients, vinegar, and zucchini and stir until smooth. Add walnuts and stir well. Pour batter into the loaf pan and bake for 45 minutes.

3. Slice and serve.

Nutrition: Calories 78, Carbs 4.4g, Fat 5.8g, Protein 3.4g

36. Tangy Barbecue Tofu Pizza

Preparation time: 20 minutes

Cooking time: 2 hours

Servings: 6

Ingredients:

- 12 inch of frozen whole-wheat pizza crust, thawed
- 1 cup of tofu pieces
- 1 small red onion, peeled and sliced
- 1/4 cup of chopped cilantro
- 1 1/2 teaspoons of salt
- 3/4 teaspoon of ground black pepper
- 1 tablespoon of olive oil
- 1 cup of barbecue sauce
- 2 cups of vegan mozzarella

Directions:

1. Place a large non-stick skillet pan over an average heat, add 1 tablespoon of oil and let it heat.
2. Add the tofu pieces in a single layer sprinkle it with 1 teaspoon of salt, black pepper and cook for 5 to 7 minutes or until it gets crispy with a golden brown on all sides.
3. Transfer the tofu pieces into a bowl, add 1/2 cup of the barbecue sauce and toss it properly to coat.

4. Grease a 4 to 6 quarts slow cooker with a non-stick cooking spray and insert the pizza crust in it.
5. Press the dough into the bottom and spread the remaining 1/2 cup of the barbecue sauce.
6. Evenly garnish it with tofu pieces and onion slices.
7. Sprinkle it with the mozzarella cheese and cover it with the lid.
8. Plug in the slow cooker and let it cook for 1 to 1 1/2 hours at the low heat setting or until the crust turns golden brown.
9. When done, transfer the pizza into the cutting board, let it rest for 10 minutes and slice to serve.

Nutrition: Calories: 135 Cal, Carbohydrates: 15g, Protein: 6g, Fats: 5g, Fiber: 1g.

SOUP AND STEW

37. African Pineapple Peanut Stew

Preparation Time: 10 minutes

Cooking Time: 20 minutes

Servings: 4

Ingredients:

- 4 cups sliced kale
- 1 cup chopped onion
- 1/2 cup peanut butter
- 1 tbsp. hot pepper sauce or 1 tbsp. Tabasco sauce
- 2 minced garlic cloves
- 1/2 cup chopped cilantro
- 2 cups pineapple, undrained, canned & crushed
- 1 tbsp. vegetable oil

Directions:

1. In a saucepan (preferably covered), sauté the garlic and onions in the oil until the onions are lightly browned, approximately 10 minutes, stirring often.
2. Wash the kale, till the time the onions are sauté.

3. Get rid of the stems. Mound the leaves on a cutting surface & slice crosswise into slices (preferably 1" thick).

4. Now put the pineapple and juice to the onions & bring to a simmer. Stir the kale in, cover and simmer until just tender, stirring frequently, approximately 5 minutes.

5. Mix in the hot pepper sauce, peanut butter & simmer for more 5 minutes.

6. Add salt according to your taste.

Nutrition: kcal: 402 Carbohydrates: 7 g Protein: 21 g Fat: 34 g

38. Vegetable Broth Sans Sodium

Preparation Time: 5 minutes

Cooking Time: 60 minutes

Servings: 1 cup

Ingredients:

- 5 sprigs of dill
- 2 freshly sliced yellow onions
- 4 chives
- 6 freshly peeled and sliced carrots
- 10 cups of water
- 4 freshly sliced celery stalks
- 3 cloves of freshly minced garlic
- 4 sprigs of parsley

Directions:

1. Put a large pot on medium heat and stir the onions. Fry the onions for 1 minute until they become fragrant. Add the garlic, celery, carrots, and dill along with the chives and parsley and cook everything. You will know that the mix is ready when it becomes fragrant.
2. Add the water and allow the mixture to boil. Reduce the heat and allow everything to cook for 45 minutes.
3. Turn off the heat. The broth will cool in about 15 minutes.

4. Strain the broth with the help of a sieve so that you have a clear vegetable broth.
5. If you are not using the broth right away, store it as ice cubes. You can store the ice cubes for a week.

Nutrition: kcal: 362 Carbohydrates: 21 g Protein: 12 g Fat: 21 g

SAUCES, DRESSINGS & DIP

39. Pistachio Dip

Preparation time: 10 minutes

Cooking time: 10 minutes

Servings: 8

Ingredients:

- 2 tablespoon lemon juice
- 1 t. extra virgin olive oil
- 2 tablespoons of the following:
- Tahini
- Parsley, chopped
- 2 cloves of garlic
- 1/2 c. pistachios shelled
- 15 oz. garbanzo beans, save the liquid from the can
- Salt and pepper to taste

Directions:

1. Using a food processor, add pistachios, pepper, sea salt, lemon juice, olive oil, tahini, parsley, garlic, and garbanzo beans. Pulse until mixed.

2. Using the liquid from the garbanzo beans, add to the dip while slowly blending until it reaches your desired consistency.

3. Enjoy at room temperature or warmed.

Nutrition: Calories: 88 Carbohydrates: 9 g Proteins: 2.5 g Fats: 3 g

40. Smokey Tomato Jam

Preparation time: 45 minutes

Cooking time: 45 minutes

Servings: 1 cup

Ingredients:

- 1/2 t. of the following:
- White wine vinegar
- Salt
- 1/3 t. smoked paprika
- Pinch Black pepper
- 1/4 c. coconut sugar
- 2 pounds' tomatoes

Directions:

1. Over medium-high heat, bring a big pot of water to a boil.
2. Fill a big bowl with ice and water.
3. Carefully place the tomatoes into the boiling water for 1 minute and then remove, and immediately put into the ice water.
4. While tomatoes are in the ice water, peel them by hand and then transfer to a clean cutting surface.

5. Empty the pot of water.

6. Chop the tomatoes and place back into the pot; add the coconut sugar and stir to combine.

7. Bring the pot back to medium heat and the tomatoes to a boil, cooking for 15 minutes.

8. Stir in the paprika, pepper, and salt and then bring the temperature down to the lowest setting. Let it cook until it becomes thick, which is approximately 10 minutes.

9. Remove it from the heat while continuing to stir; add in white wine vinegar.

Nutrition: Calories: 26 Carbohydrates: 5.3 g Proteins: 1.1 g Fats: 0.6 g

APPETIZER

41. Garden Patch Sandwiches on Multigrain Bread

Preparation time: 15 minutes

Cooking time: 0 minutes

Servings: 4

Ingredients:

- 1pound extra-firm tofu, drained and patted dry
- 1 medium red bell pepper, finely chopped
- 1 celery rib, finely chopped
- 3 green onions, minced
- ¼ cup shelled sunflower seeds
- ½ cup vegan mayonnaise, homemade or store-bought
- ½ teaspoon salt
- ½ teaspoon celery salt
- ¼ teaspoon freshly ground black pepper
- 8 slices whole grain bread
- 4 (¼-inch) slices ripe tomato
- 4 lettuce leaves

Directions:

1. Crumble your tofu then place it in a large bowl. Add the bell pepper, celery, green onions, and sunflower seeds. Stir in the mayonnaise, salt, celery salt, and pepper and mix until well combined.

2. Toast the bread, if desired. Spread the mixture evenly onto 4 slices of the bread. Put on top the tomato slice, lettuce leaf, and the remaining bread. Slice the sandwiches diagonally in half then serve.

Nutrition: Calories: 130 Carbs: 17g Fat: 7g Protein: 2g

42. Garden Salad Wraps

Preparation time: 15 minutes

Cooking time: 10 minutes

Servings: 4

Ingredients:

- 6 tablespoons extra-virgin olive oil
- 1-pound extra-firm tofu, drained, patted dry, and cut into ½-inch strips
- 1 tablespoon soy sauce
- ¼ cup apple cider vinegar
- 1 teaspoon yellow or spicy brown mustard
- ½ teaspoon salt
- ¼ teaspoon freshly ground black pepper
- 3 cups shredded romaine lettuce
- 3 ripe Roma tomatoes, finely chopped
- 1 large carrot, shredded
- 1 medium English cucumber, peeled and chopped
- 1/3 cup minced red onion
- ¼ cup sliced pitted green olives
- 4 (10-inch) whole-grain flour tortillas or lavash flatbread

Directions:

1. Warm-up 2 tablespoons of the oil in a large skillet over medium heat. Add the tofu and cook until golden brown. Sprinkle with soy sauce and set aside to cool.

2. In a small bowl, combine the vinegar, mustard, salt and pepper with the remaining 4 tablespoons oil, stirring to blend well. Set aside.

3. Combine the lettuce, tomatoes, carrot, cucumber, onion, and olives in a large bowl. Put on the dressing then toss to coat.

4. To assemble wraps, place 1 tortilla on a work surface and spread with about one-quarter of the salad. Place a few strips of tofu on the tortilla and roll up tightly. Slice in half.

Nutrition: Calories: 85 Carbs: 17g Fat: 0g Protein: 46g

43. Black Sesame Wonton Chips

Preparation time: 5 minutes

Cooking time: 5 minutes

Servings: 24 chips

Ingredients:

- 12 Vegan Wonton Wrappers
- Toasted sesame oil
- 1/3 cup black sesame seeds
- Salt

Directions:

1. Preheat the oven to 450°F. Oil a baking sheet then set aside. Cut the wonton wrappers in half crosswise, oiled them with sesame oil, then arrange them in a single layer on your prepared baking sheet.

2. Sprinkle wonton wrappers with the sesame seeds and salt. Bake until crisp and golden brown. Cool completely before serving.

Nutrition: Calories: 180 Carbs: 31g Fat: 1g Protein: 10g

SMOOTHIES AND JUICES

44. <u>Fruit Infused Water</u>

Preparation time: 5 minutes

Cooking time: 0 minute

Servings: 2

Ingredients:

- 3 strawberries, sliced
- 5 mint leaves
- ½ of orange, sliced
- 2 cups of water

Directions:

1. Divide fruits and mint between two glasses, pour in water, stir until just mixed, and refrigerate for 2 hours.
2. Serve straight away.

Nutrition: Calories: 5.4 Cal Fat: 0.1 g Carbs: 1.3 g Protein: 0.1 g Fiber: 0.4 g

45. Hazelnut and Chocolate Milk

Preparation time: 5 minutes

Cooking time: 0 minute

Servings: 2

Ingredients:

- 2 tablespoons cocoa powder
- 4 dates, pitted
- 1 cup hazelnuts
- 3 cups of water

Direction:

1. Place all the ingredients in the order in a food processor or blender and then pulse for 2 to 3 minutes at high speed until smooth.
2. Pour the smoothie into two glasses and then serve.

Nutrition: Calories: 120 Cal Fat: 5 g Carbs: 19 g Protein: 2 g Fiber: 1 g

DESSERTS

46. Orange and Cranberry Quinoa Bites

Preparation time: 25 minutes

Cooking time: 0 minutes

Servings: 12

Ingredients:

- 2 tablespoons almond butter
- 2 tablespoons maple syrup (optional)
- Zest of 1 orange
- 1 tablespoon dried cranberries
- ¾ cup cooked quinoa
- ¼ cup ground almonds
- 1 tablespoon chia seeds
- ¼ cup sesame seeds, toasted
- ½ teaspoon vanilla extract

Directions:

1. Mix the almond butter and maple syrup (if desired) in a medium bowl until smooth. Stir in the remaining ingredients, and mix to hold together in a ball.

2. Divide and form the mixture into 12 balls. Put them on a baking sheet lined with parchment paper. Put in the fridge to set for about 15 minutes. Serve chilled.

Nutrition: Calories: 109 Fat: 11.0g Carbs: 5.0g Protein: 3.0g

47. Orange Glazed Bananas

Preparation time: 15 minutes

Cooking time: 4 minutes

Servings: 6-8

Ingredients:

- 1/3 cup fresh orange juice
- 6 ripe bananas, peeled and sliced
- 1 teaspoon vanilla extract
- ½ teaspoon ground cinnamon

Directions:

1. Put the orange juice in a saucepan and warm over medium heat. Add the sliced bananas and cook for 2 minutes.
2. Add the vanilla and cinnamon and continue to cook until the moisture is absorbed, about another 2 minutes. Serve warm.

Nutrition: Calories: 98 Fat: 0.4g Carbs: 24.7g Protein: 1.2g

48. **Pear Squares**

Preparation time: 40 minutes

Cooking time: 50 minutes

Servings: 24 squares

Ingredients:

Filling:

- 1 (1-pound) can pears, with juice
- 2 cups chopped dried pears
- ¾ cup pitted dates
- ¼ cup tapioca
- 1 teaspoon orange extract

Crust:

- ½ cup pitted dates
- 1½ cups water
- ½ cup whole-wheat flour
- 1½ cups regular rolled oats
- 1/8 teaspoon salt (optional)
- 1 teaspoon vanilla extract

Topping:

- 1 cup regular rolled oats

Directions:

1. Put the canned pears and juice in a food processor and process until puréed. Transfer to a saucepan. Add the dried pears, dates, and tapioca. Simmer, covered, for 20 minutes. Add the orange extract and set aside.

2. Warm your oven to 375°F. Combine the dates plus water in a food processor and process until finely ground.

3. In a bowl, combine the date water (reserve ¼ cup), flour, oats, salt (if desired), and vanilla. Press into a baking dish and bake for 10 minutes.

4. Meanwhile, toss the remaining rolled oats with the reserved date water. Spoon the filling over the crust. Sprinkle, the oat topping over the filling.

5. Bake in the preheated oven within 20 minutes, or until firm. Cool and cut into 2-inch squares before serving.

Nutrition: Calories: 112 Fat: 0.8g Carbs: 27.5g Protein: 2.2g

49.   Prune, Grapefruit, and Orange Compote

Preparation time: 15 minutes

Cooking time: 4 minutes

Servings: 4

Ingredients:

- 1 cup pitted prunes
- ¾ cup fresh orange juice
- 1 tablespoon maple syrup (optional)
- 2 (1-pound) cans unsweetened grapefruit sections, drained
- 2 (11-ounce) cans unsweetened mandarin oranges, drained

Directions:

1. Put the prunes, orange juice, and maple syrup (if desired) in a saucepan. Bring to a boil, reduce the heat, and cook gently for 1 minute. Remove from the heat and cool.
2. Combine the mixture with the grapefruit and mandarin oranges.

3. Stir to mix. Cover and refrigerate for at least 2 hours before serving.

Nutrition: Calories: 303 Fat: 0.7g Carbs: 77.2g Protein: 4.3g

50. Pumpkin Pie Squares

Preparation time: 15 minutes

Cooking time: 30 minutes

Servings: 16 squares

Ingredients:

- 1 cup unsweetened almond milk
- 1 teaspoon vanilla extract
- 7 ounces dates, pitted and chopped
- 1¼ cups old-fashioned rolled oats
- 2 teaspoons pumpkin pie spice
- 1 (15-ounce) can pure pumpkin

Directions:

1. Warm your oven to 375°F (190°C). Put the parchment paper in a baking pan. Stir together the milk and vanilla in a bowl. Soak the dates in it for 15 minutes, or until the dates become softened.

2. Add the rolled oats to a food processor and pulse the oats into flour. Remove the oat flour from the food processor bowl and whisk together with the pumpkin pie spice in a different bowl.

3. Place the milk mixture into the food processor and process until smooth. Add the flour mixture and pumpkin to the food processor and pulse until the

mixture has broken down into a chunky paste consistency.

4. Transfer the batter to the prepared pan and smooth the top with a silicone spatula. Bake within 30 minutes, or until a toothpick inserted in the center of the pie comes out clean. Let cool completely before cutting into squares. Serve cold.

Nutrition: Calories: 68 Fat: 0.9g Carbs: 16.8g Protein: 2.3g

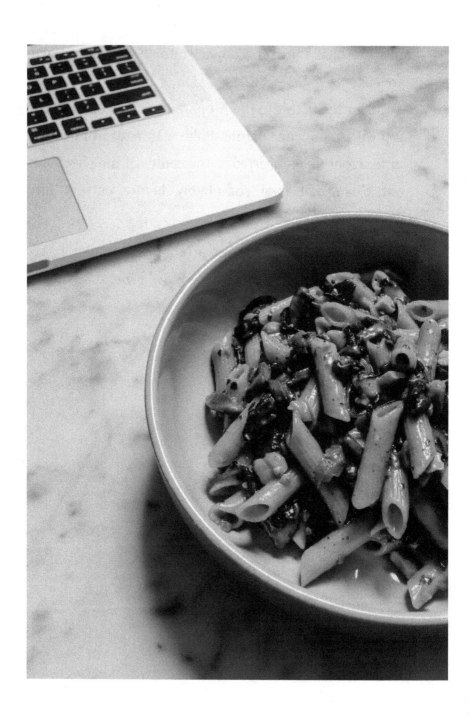

CPSIA information can be obtained
at www.ICGtesting.com
Printed in the USA
BVHW092152220421
605633BV00004B/853

9 781801 832700